The Health Benefits of Adrenal Metabolism

How to save and strengthen your adrenal glands

Dr. Cass Ingram

Knowledge House Publishers

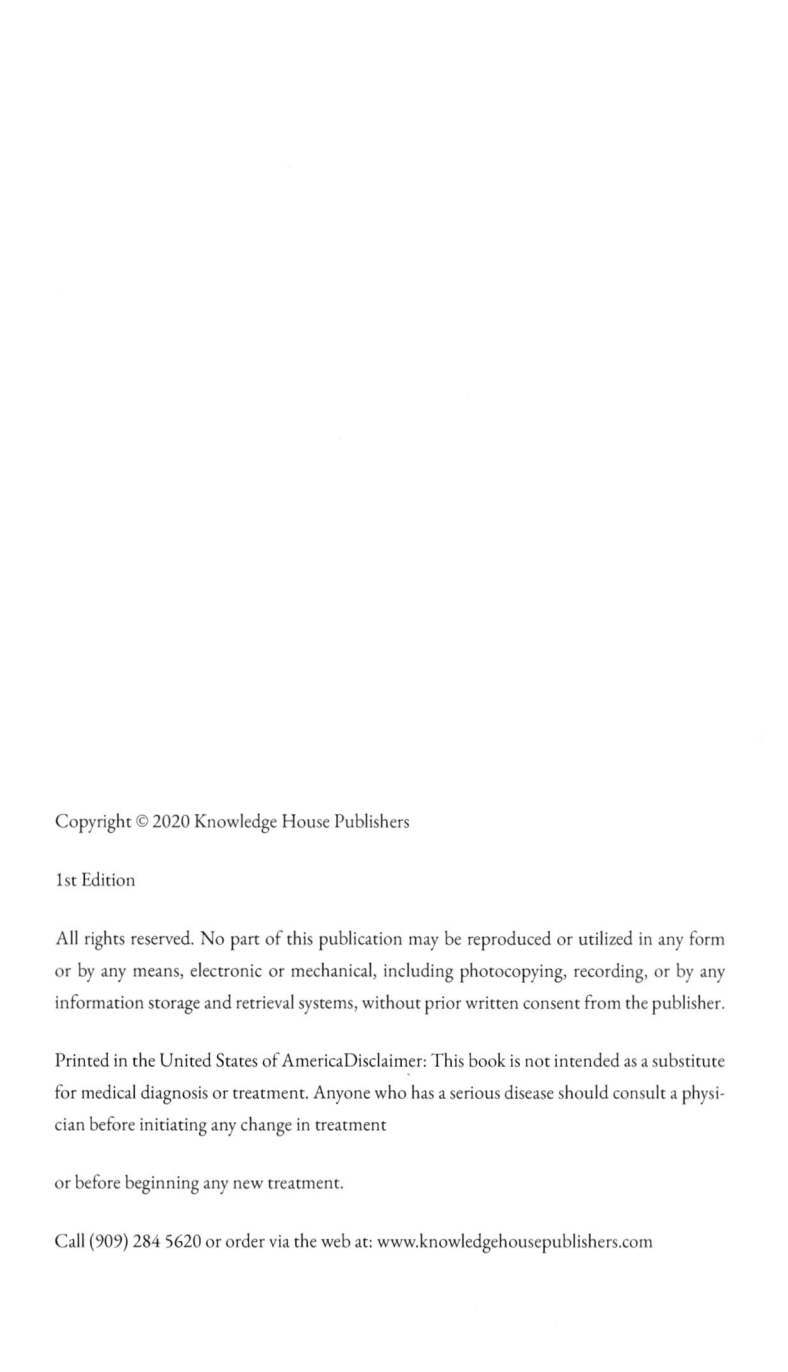

Copyright © 2020 Knowledge House Publishers

1st Edition

All rights reserved. No part of this publication may be reproduced or utilized in any form or by any means, electronic or mechanical, including photocopying, recording, or by any information storage and retrieval systems, without prior written consent from the publisher.

Printed in the United States of AmericaDisclaimer: This book is not intended as a substitute for medical diagnosis or treatment. Anyone who has a serious disease should consult a physician before initiating any change in treatment

or before beginning any new treatment.

Call (909) 284 5620 or order via the web at: www.knowledgehousepublishers.com

Contents

1. Introduction   1
2. A dietary disease?   5
3. What is an Adrenal Type?   12
4. Diet and Therapy   21
5. Vulnerabilities   29
6. Testing Yourself   34
7. Vaccination: aSerious Assault   39
8. Conclusion   42

About the Author   46

Chapter One

Introduction

The adrenal glands are one of the most crucial of all human organ systems. These delicate organs are the main coping mechanism of the body. Tiny yet powerful the adrenals are forced into action with any stress or toxicity, whether mental, chemical, or physical. There are two of them, situated atop each kidney. It was found in the 1930s that if one was surgically removed, typically, the patient died. Now, if this was to occur, people are kept alive through artificial hormone replacement. Contrast this to the kidneys, where it is possible that a person could function adequately on only 30% of function.

These glands play a crucial role in healthy food metabolism and digestion. They are also key for circulation, blood sugar control, salt balance, muscular strength, and immunity. How such a miniscule organ could control such critical and extensive functions is astonishing to say the least. To further demonstrate their importance the adrenal glands make nearly 70 hormones, all of which operate on the innermost mechanisms of the body.

With, perhaps, the richest blood and nerve supply of any organ this demonstrates their crucial importance. This organ system comprises an inner portion, or medulla, and the outer, the cortex. The inside makes adrenalin, while the outer part produces a wide range of specialized hormones, known as adrenal steroids. This book will focus on the cortex and the role of its impressive production of these hormones in human health. In fact, by definition the adrenal body type it is one in which the adrenal cortex is insufficient.

To illustrate the importance of this system it has a rich blood supply, one of the most profuse in all the body. It is also extensively supplied with nerves, primarily from the sympathetic nervous system. In fact, it has a denser supply of nerves than the kidneys themselves on which these organs sit atop.

The adrenals are responsible for the so-called fight or flight syndrome, which is based upon dealing with threats or crises of all types. In those with the sluggish adrenal type the ability to handle stress-like crises is greatly diminished. This includes physical stresses, like sudden infections, accidents, and vaccinations.

Continuously, people report that they feel their adrenals are an issue. Saying they are "run down," such individuals are unable to handle any degree of stress or pressure. Further psychic impositions would cause them to go into a downward spiral, to virtually collapse. Clearly, they cannot cope. Thus, they lack all adrenal reserve. Others say that they are weak with no stamina and that their muscles have no strength or tone. Still others complain of blood sugar imbalances: lightheadedness, fatigue, dizziness, fainting spells, irritability, and more. Seemingly, everyone with adrenal exhaustion complains that stress negatively impacts them and that they can't handle any further burdens. In contrast, hard work seems to be well-tolerated, as long as it isn't associated with mental duress.

Though their nervous systems are under siege and, therefore, they love private time adrenal types can do fine as long as they are left alone. It is not that they are antisocial, far from the case. It is just that they can't handle being tormented, especially psychologically. Attempts by intolerant ones to impose their will upon them, making extraordinary demands, putting pressure upon pressure, causes them such strain that, emotionally, they literally fall apart. Simply put, they lack sufficient cortisol to sufficiently fight back.

There are circulatory disturbances, notably cold hands and feet as well as low blood pressure. Because of an imbalance in electrolytes there is little desire to drink water or other fluids. Simultaneously, there usually is a great craving for salt.

There is also the common complaint of disorders related to the nerves. The condition may lead to many mental and neurological problems, which may range from mild to extreme. These include anxiety, nervousness, agitation, and depression. Yet, it can also lead to obsessive-compulsive behavior, psychosis, neurosis, and even schizophrenia.

In truly extreme cases the mental disarray can be dramatic. Because of the seriousness of the symptoms in many instances antidepressants and also antipsychotics are prescribed. There are in some cases temper fits and psychotic behavior that drive a person to be hospitalized and/or institutionalized. This is from adrenal dysfunction as it relates to blood sugar.

The brain relies upon glucose, the sugar of the blood, for energy. It consumes up to 80% of the body's production. In adrenal cases there is a pattern. This is the inability to consistently maintain the needed levels. In moderate and severe dysfunction a specific abnormality develops: flattening of the blood sugar levels below the optimal. As a result, the brain is unable to gain sufficient fuel. Plus, there are challenges of the fluctuations from the highs and the lows. In the latter the brain simply is virtually starved of the energy sources it so desperately requires. Nor can the muscles gain sufficient supplies to burn as fuel. This causes adrenal types to relentlessly crave sugar. Yet, when it is consumed, all this does is drive the abnormality deeper and despite intake, less sugar than before is available to the tissues. This habitual consumption exacerbates all the symptoms, often magnifying the mental incapacitation but also the fatigue and weakness. No doubt, the addiction is extreme. It may also be physiologic, like the habituation to cocaine or heroin.

They also crave salt. This may alternate; a person may eat something sugary, causing the blood sugar to be disturbed and to plummet, then eat salty food to compensate. This is because salt reduces adrenal stress, while simultaneously increasing hormone production. No one could imagine it could do this. The hormones aldosterone and the glucocorticoids are needed to manage that blood sugar level. People don't know it, but the imbalances in their organs are driving these cravings. These cravings are important symptoms for determining the seriousness of the adrenal imbalance syndrome.

How does this work in real time? When sugar or starch is consumed, it is digested and then enters the blood stream. The body reacts by secreting insulin, yet another hormone produced by the pancreas. With refined sugars and starches this forces the pancreas to over-shoot and the too high insulin levels cause the blood to fall below normal and to be erratic. Now, the adrenals must come into play. Producing the glucocorticoids their job is to manage the blood sugar, essentially, level it after the insulin sugar. If they fail to do so, there is nothing other than metabolic chaos. Yet, the minimum that must be realized is that every dose of refined sugar and starch leads to stress upon these glands by forcing an exhaustion in its synthetic abilities.

Chapter Two

A dietary disease?

Adrenal insufficiency is driven by diet more than any other factor. Until the introduction of heavily processed food it was unknown. More than any other factor it is directly related to sugar consumption. In its worst form, Addison's disease, it was discovered just after refined sugar was extensively introduced to the Western diet.

This was by conspiracy. People had typically used this only as a specialty substance, locked in the cabinet for special events: like making a holiday cake. The sugar industry, becoming robust by the 1840s, had different plans. Through schemes and plots industry operators put salesmen to work. These agents gave out in the major cities packets of sugar, causing people to become addicted. Now, they sought the sugary foods. This was in primarily England and the United States. As consumption increased, so did the incidence of Addison's disease. In fact, the disease was unknown prior to sugar's introduction.

Another factor was the introduction in the early 1900s of the roller mill. This was the means by which the germ and bran was removed from the grains, leaving only the starch. This led to the production of all manner of heavily processed foods, aggravating the adrenal insufficiency syndromes. If for no other reason than these are schemes and plots against the people, these refined food sources must be strictly avoided. This will give the adrenal glands, finally, a chance to regenerate.

Make no mistake refined sugar causes severe disruption of the adrenal glands. The body thrives on sugar, but it maintains levels tightly. When that deviant of nature refined carbohydrates are consumed, like sugar and white flour, the body initially deals with this through insulin. Once that hormone finishes its job, processing the with the spike, the hormonal controlling system comes in for the rest of the hours of blood balancing. This is via the adrenals through the glucocorticoids. These glands are unable to handle the load of refined carbohydrates, though the cells work overtime to combat this. Eventually, they become depleted. The overworked adrenals burn out and actually suffer cell death. When this happens, known as adrenal cellular necrosis, this diseased tissue becomes infected. This is typically by tuberculosis, but various fungi may play a role. Every additional dose of refined sugar further deepens the degree of infection until the victim virtually collapses; premature death may result. When Addison autopsied these cases in the 1850s, he found most of them had active tuberculosis infestation. It has not diminished. In fact, today, upon autopsy, some one of three Americans are found to have active TB in their adrenals. It is worsened in those who eat chocolate and cacao, a deliberate adrenal poison.

Most people have a much lesser degree of this. Instead of suffering from potentially fatal Addison's disease they are enduring a chronic, insidious type, which is known as "subclinical Addison's disease." The deficit or dysfunctional hormones are all produced by the adrenal cortex, thus the other descriptive term, hyoadrenalcorticism. It is known here as sluggish adrenal syndrome or adrenal insufficiency. To have this condition is a serious issue and must not be taken lightly.

Through his 1950s-era research the endocrinologist and adrenal syndrome expert John Tintera, M.D., lays this all out. Based upon 200 cases he provides a chart of all the main symptoms and signs of the syndrome. Most of these are found in the adrenal self-test found here and also online at www.purelywildnatural.com.

While Tintera coined the term originally as subclinical Addison's disease, the tests here plus the Website assessments h. For purposes of this book it will be deemed adrenal insufficiency, or exhaustion, sluggish adrenal syndrome, and 'collapse' of this system. The latter term clearly describes what is happening, that because of this incapacitation, the person is unable to cope.

Let us at least list what he determined to be the essential, primary symptoms. These include the following in order of frequency:

- fatigue
- nervousness
- cravings for salt
- inability to concentrate
- cravings for sweets
- irritability
- depression
- apprehension
- excessive weakness
- headache
- palpitations

Anyone who suffers with at least three of these has a chronic case of adrenal insufficiency. Most of these symptoms are likely a result of the blood sugar disorders, which are ultra-common in this syndrome. These are the symptoms of hypoglycemia, and this demonstrates how critical are the adrenals in blood sugar control.

It is the emotions, said Tintera, that often provoke adrenal-related blood sugar imbalances. Emotional stress is accompanied with the release of nerve impulses that can lead to the secretion of insulin. This then results in a drop in blood sugar levels, which motivates the adrenal glands to produce antagonistic hormones. In chronic cases they may be unable to do so. Without sound function of these glands as a back-up to the pancreas the blood sugar drops excessively and remain low. This is complicated in the event of liver dysfunction, since this organ is also heavily involved in blood sugar maintenance.

Like the adrenals the liver is readily disturbed by excessive carbohydrate consumption, especially the ingestion of refined sugar. Corn sweeteners and alcohol also readily corrupt it, and white flour is also disruptive. Their consumption inevitably leads to fatty liver and thus its degeneration. As a storage and release depot it plays a heavy role in glucose metabolism and is directly involved in any blood sugar upsets endured by the adrenals. The site for storing and releasing glycogen the substance acts as a critical emergency food for supplying the body's struggling needs.

As harsh as the refined carbohydrates are it readily accepts natural sugar complexes such as raw honey and coconut sugar. Whole fruit is also well-tolerated. Adrenal cases handle most fruit readily, although in extreme cases even this may have to be restricted.

For adrenal insufficiency diet is the key. As soon as modifications in the diet are made the symptoms often dramatically improve. Think of it this way. Refined sugar and starch directly and immediately forces these two organs into disarray. In contrast, naturally fat-rich food, such as butter, cream, avocadoes, and similar dietary items, greatly nourish it. The same is true of high-protein sources such as eggs and grass-fed meat. The point is none of these food sources create blood sugar spikes and therefore lead to the outpouring of hormones. Essentially, eating them, especially when using salt, rests the glands.

Another source of this resting is fasting, though not all adrenal cases readily tolerate this, because of the flattening of their blood sugar curves. Even so, by not bombarding the body with food or drink it has a chance to regenerate. Also, fasting aids in the rebuilding of the intestinal lining and the detoxification of the liver as well as the kidneys. The ideal fast is the Islamic type where no food or drink is taken, basically from an hour or so before sunrise all the way to sunset.

The Mind and the Adrenals

The state of the mind plays a vast role in adrenal health. While all this has already been alluded to this section serves as an in-depth analysis of the connection.

It is highly simplistic. An upbeat, positive attitude boosts adrenal health. In contrast, a negative, dour one devastates it. To maintain optimal status it is critical to maintain that positivity. Not for a moment can a person fall into destructive thinking. That type of thinking is so devastating that it can immediately lead to a degree of ruination of health.

There is a secretive power to this. That is almost being amused with life. It is to be amused with your own self and never to take life or events too seriously. Maintaining the right overall attitude, in fact, is so important an entire book could be written about it. The crucialness is so great that it is equal to sound nutrition and healthy exercise.

Adrenal types know this well. Typically, they go through bouts of thinking in a self-deprecating way. Allowing in worry, guilt, and frustration, first-hand they experienced the consequences. Adrenal people know the danger. Yet, it doesn't hurt to remind.

There are certain extremely toxic thinking processes that disturb these glands. A rather complete list of these thinking and behavior patterns is as follows:

- guilt
- worry
- frustration
- anxiousness
- anger
- raising the voice and exhibiting temper tantrums
- arguing
- acting mean and hostile
- unrelenting grief
- lack of faith, agnosticism and/or godlessness

There is no means for the adrenal glands to handle these. What's more, rapidly, these emotional states deplete the glands' reserves. Guilt is perhaps the worse. Immediately, this cannibalizes adrenal capacities. If it is allowed to continue for a prolonged period, this organ system can fall into failure.

Any time there is anything but peace in the nervous system this leads to a crisis. It can be said that all non-peaceful thinking is aberrant. That means that arguing and meanness are the opposite of what the body is geared for. The same is true of guilt and remorse.

Both guilt and grieving are highly destructive to adrenal function. For an adrenal person to survive all such emotional disarray must be eliminated. The Prophet Muhammad, for one, gives guidance here. He tells people that even in the worst crisis, like the loss of a dearest loved one, the grief period is limited, like one day. The adrenals can handle this minor load. For avoidance of all hostility, arguing, and hatefulness he made an additional invaluable dictate. Each person of the faith is to greet the other with "Peace be upon you," and the return greeting, "and peace be upon you as well."

Worst of all is a virtual complete lack of faith. This is seen to a dramatic degree in those who have no belief, who actually refuse to believe in almighty God. People make that choice; they suffer emotionally for it. The agnostic, the undecided one, suffers to a degree less. What a loss it is for any such individuals, especially from an adrenal function capacity. After all, hearts do find peace, denotes the Qur'an, the holy book of Islam, in the "remembrance of God." What a simple tool to use, if people only realized it.

The refusal to believe in the divine Being is a form of hostility, even arrogance. This emotion is harsh on the adrenals; they cannot readily handle this load, that is the one of a human putting himself so high.

Humility is the opposite of this, which nourishes and relaxes the glands. The deeper is the humility and the resulting peacefulness the more powerful, also the more well-rested, these glands become. A person can easily sense the peace that humbleness produces; it virtually makes an individual smile, as such a one is connected directly to consciousness with God Himself.

A person should learn from these dictums and be a peace at all times; never allow the descent into anger. If an individual feels an element of rage, do a simple technique; sit down and relax. If there is inevitable grief, experience it short-term, then give the rest to God. Be at peace. The adrenals will respond in kind.

Chapter Three

What is an Adrenal Type?

The adrenal type is the person who was weak adrenals. In many respects it is an inherited syndrome. In utero, these individuals were lacking in the proper development of the glands and, therefore, in adrenal hormone production. Plus, as they developed in youth the deficiency was magnified, largely by wrong dietary habits. This is especially the excessive consumption of refined sugar. As well, those who were born from mothers and fathers who drank alcohol excessively frequently suffer the condition.

The syndrome is easy to diagnose based upon signs and symptoms. The basic manifestations have already been listed. Even so, people with this vulnerability have a certain look. What is that overall appearance? They are usually thin and fine-boned. Certain of them are even tall and lanky. This type has a relatively fast metabolism, and so even when eating large quantities of food rarely gains excessive weight. However, if weight is gained, it is usually in the buttocks or hips or around the lower abdomen, like at the belly-button level.

In some cases the weakness can be extreme, where they are hardly able to function. The reason for the weakness is easily explained. Steroid hormones are essential for muscular strength and also for stamina. The steroids also regulate blood sugar levels. Neither the brain nor the muscles can function without adequate blood sugar as fuel.

Adrenal types are often highly gentle. Some of them are delicate and loving, even soft and kind. They can also be extremely sensitive. This can be to the point where they become emotional wrecks. In this regard their feelings are easily hurt and they might cry readily. Often highly instinctive, adrenal types may also border on being intuitive. In some cases they may know or sense issues, such as impeding disasters, before anyone else.

With a tendency to fume or agitate excessively the adrenal personality may become somewhat paranoid. However, they can use such senses to their advantage, for instance, for clairvoyance, intuition, financial capacities, inventions, and similar productive pursuits. Even so, there are certain derogatory aspects to this sensitivity. Often, concentration is impaired. This is the person who finds it difficult to focus on important tasks. There may be a sensation which is bizarre, which is an internal nervousness. While depression is common, as is insomnia, nervousness, anxiety, and agitation are more common than depression. The anxiety can be severe, especially in those who maintain the high sugar consumption. In some cases there may be a kind of mental dullness and also confusion. These are among the mind-related symptoms determined by Tintera, which also included poor concentration, apprehension, and irritability, also emphasizing the sleeplessness. Clearly, the connection to adrenal exhaustion to normal function of the mind is profound.

<u>Main Signs</u>

There are both the symptoms, some already mentioned, but also the signs. Typically, there are certain physical characteristics, which are revealing. Many adrenal types are frail. They have a lesser bone structure than the average individual. However, the prominent feature is a receding chin. The facial bones are fine; the jaw bones especially are unusually small with all bones of the rest of the face following. The cheeks are generally not large and robust, as is typical in the thyroid type.

A receding chin is a major feature. It is identified by the failure of this boney prominence to jut beyond the level plane of the face. Typically, it will be found to be, essentially, a backwards-appearing chin instead of protruding normally forward. Because of the smaller facial bones, especially involving the jaw, the teeth develop abnormally. There is simply not enough room for them to grow. Thus, there is the finding of crowding of the teeth, especially the lower incisors. If the upper ones are also crowded upon themselves, this is a sign of extreme adrenal vulnerability. As well, the roof of the mouth is usually of diminished size and arched.

Another major issue revolves around finger length. The hand/finger sign is perhaps the easiest one to recognize. The individual often has a long index finger versus the ring—normal is when the index finger is longer. Or, the fingers may be the same length, which still indicates an adrenal propensity. When they are longer on both sides, the adrenal type is confirmed.

These anomalies are directly related to developmental vulnerabilities. The sound, normal building of bone mass is powered by the androgens. A major function of sound adrenals is to produce them. The deficit of these directly impacts the bone density profile, even leading to an elongation of the digits. A short index finger is a sign of sufficient androgen production, with a long one compared to the ring denoting severe deficiency.

There may be other physical elements which are observable. The eyes are often sunken; there may be dark circles. The coloration may include a purplish-red appearance arising from the corners of the eyes. Of note, this is a sign of parasitic infestation for which adrenal types are vulnerable. Actually, any reddish or purplish induration under the eyes is an indication of adrenal type, which reveals an intestinal disorder. If it is generalized, this is typical of allergic propensities. Anyone with sluggishness of these glands is vulnerable to gut-based food reactions.

The hair is medium-fine to fine. In men, usually, the hair on the head is thinner than normal, even if it is relatively full, although there may be male-pattern baldness; this is also common in thyroid types. Additionally, there is a tendency for it to be straight rather than curly. It may be wispy. In fact, in a blond, blue-eyed person fine, straight hair of a wispy nature is virtual proof of this type.

In the pure adrenal type the metabolism can be in all realms: medium, rapid, and slow. Some individuals are thin, others plump and pudgy, and still others overweight. The heavy-set ones have a thyroid and/or pituitary component, although they may also be infested with fungus. The fungus causes them to be bloated and to retain fluid, especially if in reaction to sugar consumption.

Demonstrating another element of their poor blood sugar control adrenal cases may be fuss-budgets. There may also be the habit of nervous agitation. They may be seen to be pillorying, that is twisting paper or plastic into rolls and/or doing so with their hair. There may be uncontrollable irritation with a tendency to nervously tap their feet or shake their legs: or pacing. Inveterate worriers, they are unable to have peaceful and settled minds, not as long as they are steroid deficient. They often appear unhappy, largely because they are constantly fretting or, perhaps, fuming about their health.

According to *Organotherapy* published in the 1920s by C. W. Carrick Co., the main symptoms of adrenal deficit are fatigue or a feeling of being "run-down" and increased sensitivity to cold and/or cold extremities, low blood pressure, weak heart pulse, irregular heart beat, sluggish metabolism, constipation, sluggish digestion, reduced blood count, along with many of the symptoms already mentioned.

In untreated adrenal cases panic attacks, anxiety, compulsive behavior, and palpitations may be the leading symptoms. Thus, it is no surprise that this syndrome is often confused with a host of other diseases, including a wide range of psychological conditions. This leads to an incorrect diagnosis as well as the prescription of unnecessary, in fact, dangerous medications. It has also led to the absolutely dire. Millions of Americans have been hospitalized and even institutionalized under diagnoses of mental diseases when the entire problem was adrenal weakness. This includes people whose lives have been ruined by being permanently institutionalized in insane asylums.

The true adrenal type is sort of a weakling. These individuals are always in need of help. Their will power may be strong. However, their body fails to follow this. They are the people who have difficulty opening up a stuck car door or removing a tight jar lid. They are those who are attempting at all times to prevent added stresses, knowing they will be drained by them. The adrenal person might ask the spouse or someone else to check to see the doors are locked or they may do so themselves. It is all because of the preemptive attempt to avoid the stress of a theft—or simply the stress of thinking about it.

It takes little to destabilize such a person. A mere emotional reaction to a major or minor issue can devastate the adrenal case. If tremendous pressure is placed upon them, they collapse, sleeping to recover. This is far from a psychological issue; rather, it is strictly physical, that is the diminished ability to cope due to weakened adrenal function. The individual is unable to mount a sufficient adrenal response for the body to cope. Being run down, suffering the inability to cope, being excessively nervous, craving sugar and salt, and having difficulty focusing; these are major giveaways that virtually prove the diagnosis.

Pigment changes: a serious sign

In a high percentage of true Addison's cases there are pigment deposits, which are tell-tale signs. These spots usually occur after the onset of the weakness. Developing on any region of the skin they may also develop on the mucous membranes. Most commonly these pigmented lesions are found on the face, neck, back of the hands, lips, anal folds, knuckles, and similar surfaces.

There may also be a generalized alteration in the color of the skin where it takes on a tan-like appearance known as bronzing. Regarded as a serious sign this may be used to make the diagnosis of Addison's disease. This bronze coloration, like the spots, is a consequence of the excessive deposition of melanin.

Vague and difficult to diagnose

The adrenal type often develops bizarre symptoms many of which doctors are unable to understand. It may take decades to make the diagnosis if ever. Yet, the symptoms are real and often devastating. It is the adrenal individual who looks relatively healthy, that is who has no overt signs of disease, but inside feels generally "lousy." Such a person complains constantly of a wide range of seemingly vague symptoms, including digestive problems, heartburn, nausea, aches, various back pains, especially in the upper mid- to lower-back, headaches, dizziness, and fatigue, in addition to the as mentioned nervousness and weakness. Adrenal types tend to be over-workers, and, often, they are compulsive. Readily becoming sugar addicts, they may alternate sugar binges with binges of eating salty snacks. Also, they may be the typical persons who must have salty snacks while not eating an excess of sweets. Adrenal types may also crave alcohol and occasionally over-indulge in it. However, alcohol usually makes them sick, so in most cases they avoid it.

Lack of a strong voice is typical of an adrenal person. Often, it is a strain to hear them. They may even have a dragging voice, which is tiresomely monotonous. Whiners, who seem to never stop complaining or nagging, frequently, they talk endlessly, and no one can speak even a word between. They may give the appearance of being nervous, even agitated or upset. Such individuals often exhibit aggravating habits, like being fidgety or the repetitive tapping of the feet. The shopkeeper who is unable to stop talking is typically hypoadrenal. Thus, their hyperactivity is a mere compensation, a sign of adrenal weakness. These people have very little coping capacity. In contrast, truly calm people who can easily cope usually have strong adrenal glands.

As mentioned, the adrenal glands are the primary organ system for fighting stress. They are responsible for warding off the ill effects of every conceivable mental and/or physical stressor. However, emotional strain is more toxic than the physical. It causes significant disruption of adrenal function. Anger is perhaps the most devastating of all mental stressors. Researchers have discovered that its negative effects on adrenal function are profound. Therefore, they must strive to remain calm, or they will destroy themselves. With worry and fretting people with adrenal insufficiency think their way into adrenal failure. Thus, it is essential that they eliminate negative thinking patterns, which is, by the way, much easier to do once the condition is properly treated.

Their inherent weak constitution may cause them problems when growing up. In fact, they may be subjected to much during those vulnerable years. So-called bullies may readily seek them out. Even later in life, if joining with the wrong person, they may be tormented. The fact is the adrenal type is regarded by others as weak, that is physically, and so unable to defend himself/herself. Yet, actually, adrenal types are often capable of defending themselves. However, they only do so in life-threatening circumstances.

Many adrenal types have a refined, almost sophisticated, appearance. Often, they are physically and emotionally usually delicate. With their heightened perceptive ability they may sense the odor of a fire or chemical spill before any other. Their reaction to sound is abnormally acute, where they may experience a 100,000-infold increase over normal. Such an acute sensation capacity surely explains the abnormally hypersensitivity mentally, physically, and emotionally.

Determining your type

With the adrenal type there is also a tendency to develop chronic infections. In particular, there is an unusual propensity for viral lung infections. There is also a high tendency for bacterial lung infections as well as fungal infections of the lungs and bronchial tubes. These are the individuals who readily develop chronic bronchitis and asthma. The high risk for the development of tuberculosis is especially the case with wrong diet. Yet, once again, it is primarily sugar and chocolate which do so, although caffeine can be an aggravator. In this compromised state the resistance against such subtle, pervasive invaders is virtually nil. The average American consumption of refined sugar in its various forms is as much as 150 pounds per person per year. No wonder nearly accounts for the finding on autopsy in people who die of adrenal failure of TB infection actually in the glands. The question is does the TB cause the adrenal collapse, or is it an opportunist invading the glands once they are weakened?

Thus, it becomes apparent that, again, knowledge is empowering. By understanding the attributes and vulnerable aspects of their body types, the individual can take the appropriate precautions.

Chapter Four

Diet and Therapy

With the true adrenal types the treatment is relatively basic. This treatment consists of an approach for three different categories: mild, moderate, and extreme. It seems that most cases fall into the moderate-to-extreme categories. So, let us being here. The diet in these cases is a low carbohydrate one, the purpose being to take the stress off the role of the glands to manage blood sugar. This type of diet will also correct blood sugar disorders. The other arena is to avoid the excessive intake of alkaline foods, especially dark green leafy vegetables. Next is to increase the consumption of salt and salty food/snacks. Finally, it is to consume nutrient dense foods rich in fat, as this will help level blood sugar.

The diet is based upon sound physiology. It basically eliminates carbohydrate sources that are rapidly digested and absorbed, leading to blood sugar disturbances. In these moderate and extreme cases people know that these types of sugars and starches, while possibly providing a temporary positive effect, long-term, lead to all sorts of problems, including drops in blood sugar, dizziness, headaches, irritability, muscle cramps, depression, and anxiety. Nevertheless, the elimination of the food-induced excessive rise and fall of blood sugar will always result in significant improvement.

This does not mean, though, that all carbohydrates must be eliminated. Natural sources of sugars, for instance, may be tolerated such as coconut sugar, raw, wild honey, and many of the less sweet fruit such as melons and strawberries.

Anti-adrenal insufficiency diet

Foods allowed:

- All fresh, grass-fed, and organic red meats (except pork)
- Fresh, organic, or free-range poultry with the skin on
- Fresh, organic, or free-range eggs
- Whole, organic milk
- Cheese of all types
- Organic yogurt (full-fat varieties without added sugar)
- Butter
- Coconut and red palm oils
- Avocado and extra virgin olive oils

Snacks

- salted nuts and nut butter
- whole grain gluten-free crackers, salted

Fruits

- melons, papayas, kiwi, grapefruit, lemon, lime,

- blueberries, strawberries, raspberries, blackberries

- skins of apples and pears, coconut,

Starches

Quinina, teff, buckwheat, rice bran, oat brain

Top Vegetables

- Squash, artichokes, avocados, capers, broccoli, Brussels sprouts,

- cabbage, kohlrabi, sweet peppers, tomatoes, radishes, turnips,

- parsley roots, parsley, Note: if dark leafy greens are to be eaten,

Much fat needs to be added and they must be extensively salted.

Beverages

- weak tea, herbal teas, unsweetened vinegar drinks, tomato juice,

- lemon juice, grapefruit juice, wild chaga tea.

Note: orange juice, with its high glycemic index, is typically too sweet.

Supplements

- royal jelly with wild rosemary oil

- sage

- ashwagandha extract

- spice oil extracts mix containing oils of wild myrtle, plus cumin, cinnamon, fenugreek, and wild oregano. This com-

plex researched at Georgetown University, Washington, D.
C., was found to dramatically reduce blood sugar. In animals
reared as diabetics as reported in the *Journal Molecules and
Chemistry, 2001*. A near 50% reduction in blood sugar levels
was achieved in one dose.

The cholesterol issue

Forcibly lowering the cholesterol in adrenal types is a bad idea.
This is a critical nutrient for these glands. They concentrate it out
of the blood. When cut open surgically, there is a noticeable yellow
appearance with the deposition of an obvious wax. This is cholesterol,
the base material for the synthesis of all adrenal steroids. To deny it
this is to stop it from adequately producing the hormones the body
requires.

All cholesterol-lowering drugs are contraindicated in adrenal insufficiency. Clearly, the destruction of this molecule will impair glandular function, as all the key hormones, like cortisol, DHEA and testosterone, are derived from it.

Synthesizing your own hormones

To make adrenal steroids certain nutrients are required. Who would
have thought? The main ones are cholesterol and salt. For vitamins it
is primarily pantothenic acid and vitamin C but also riboflavin.

There is another critical factor, the metabolically efficient B vitamin, pantothenic acid. This vitamin is the key one for stimulating cholesterol synthesis. Without it, cholesterol production throughout the body declines and, ultimately, stalls. Top sources of this nutrient include nuts and seeds, avocados, germs of grains, red meat, dark meat of poultry, and eggs.

Meat and eggs are also rich in riboflavin, yet another substance
direly needed by the adrenal glands. This vitamin, which is commonly

deficient in the American diet, is needed for oxygen delivery within cells. In the adrenal glands it serves to speed the synthesis of cholesterol; it is an essential part of the step-wise creation of this molecule. Riboflavin keeps the oxygen metabolism within the adrenal glands in ideal condition. Thus, it is crucial for the health of this organ. Without it, oxygen metabolism in these glands is disrupted, which can lead to a decline in adrenal hormone synthesis. In the extreme the lack of riboflavin places the adrenal cells at a high risk. Oxygen can no longer be efficiently metabolized. As a result toxic forms of oxygen are produced. Steroid hormones can no longer be efficiently synthesized. The result is cell damage and death. Top sources of riboflavin are primarily animal foods, particularly organ meats, red meats, whole milk products, and eggs, although avocados contain lesser but significant amounts. Thus, diets which restrict the aforementioned foods lead to riboflavin deficiency.

High-sodium foods

In many respects a vegetable-based diet is the wrong approach in this condition. As a rule vegetation is too high in potassium, while excessively low in sodium. Such a mineral ratio causes great stress upon the adrenals, leading to the depletion of the salt-saving hormone aldosterone. In contrast, meat is high in sodium, as well as chloride, while relatively low in potassium. It has the ideal sodium/chloride to potassium ratio. Thus, it fails to weaken adrenal status, rather, strengthens it. Therefore, fresh red meat, the richest source of sodium and chloride salts, is the ideal adrenal-replenishing food. For vegans and vegetarians with adrenal syndrome it is critical to use sea salt on food liberally, but they should use only the unbleached type. This increased intake will minimize salt loss, which is inevitable on such diets. Also, such individuals should take wild-source triple salt capsules with each meal. Additionally, celery and celery root are high in sodium and would be preferred vegetables for adrenal health.

People with depleted adrenal glands may gain great strength from reasonable quantities of red meat, including organic grass-fed beef, bison, elk, venison, antelope, and similar foods. These foods give them a fairly prolonged degree of stamina, usually for hours. Poultry and fish are also ideal but not as powerful as red meat. Usually, a 10- to 12-ounce steak gives such person a great sense of strength.

Red meat contains yet another critical adrenal component. This is cholesterol. Thus, this food is a complete one for these glands, as it contains the three most critical substances, which replenish it: cholesterol, sodium, and chloride.

If eating dark greens, be sure to salt them aggressively. For instance, here is how to make spinach for the adrenal insufficient. Cook it, and drain the water (this eliminates a considerable amount of potassium). Reheat it again in a small amount of water, and discard the juice. Then, add salted butter and extra sea salt. Or, make creamed spinach using real cream (no wheat flour) plus added sea salt. This will convert the spinach from adrenal-toxic to adrenal-nourishing.

Salt: an adrenal regenerative?

The consumption of salt is crucial for re-building and also maintaining adrenal health. Fishbein claims in his medical encyclopedia that sodium loss is a critical factor in the cause of the typical symptoms of adrenal collapse, which are fatigue, weakness, and other vague symptoms. A high intake of sodium with a low intake of potassium, is the crucial formula for medicating these glands. This would imply the need to restrict the intake of high potassium foods, while instead consuming those foods relatively low in this mineral or which at least have the counteracting tissue salts. Low-potassium foods include red meat, eggs, cheese, whole milk, yogurt, quark, kefir, butter, poultry, seafood, fish, and organ meats. What's more, all such foods are relatively high in salts.

Vinegar is an adrenal tonic

Vinegar is concentrated acetic acid. This is precisely the substance needed by the body to make cholesterol. The adrenals, as well as the gonads, make cholesterol from acetic acid, known medically as acetate. Thus, by supplying acetate in the form of vinegar steroid synthesis can be boosted. It is a simple equation: supply the body with the raw materials it needs, and let it heal itself. Thus, vinegar can be used on the adrenal gland regenerative diet, but, once again, neutralize the potassium by adding salt.

Chocolate: a deadly poison?

One of the harshest foods for adrenal health is chocolate. This includes all its forms, including the now heavily trending raw cacao. The only exception is cocoa butter, which has no derogatory effect. The reason for the toxicity is a stimulant chemical virtually exclusive to chocolate, known as theobromine. An irritant, there is no way a sensitive adrenal case can handle large or even moderate amounts.

The substance, an alkaloid, has a long history of causing untoward reactions. As a rule, its consumption leads to agitation, restlessness, insomnia, and anxiety. This is largely a result of the depletion of adrenal hormones, which are secreted to deal with it. Overall, what it does is to, like caffeine, overstimulate the nervous system, and the adrenal glands must react in compensation. It is also theobromine which is the addictive substance in the cocoa bean. The bottom line is that regular and even relatively low-level consumption will fatigue the adrenal glands, worsening the adrenal type's health.

What about caffeine?

How can the consumption of a known irritating substance that rachets up the nervous system cause anything other than significant harm? By no means should adrenal types be consuming stimulants. Even the supposedly antioxidant-rich chocolate often poses an issue. High caffeine foods and beverages include the following:

- black tea
- green tea
- coffee
- chocolate
- energy drinks
- certain weight loss supplements
- certain prescription drugs
- street drugs, like cocaine and heroin

All these substances/beverages disrupt adrenal function. The stimulants act as agitators. While there may be a temporary sense of benefit, long-term the results can be devastating. The approach is basic enough. It is to simply eliminate all such foods, supplements, and beverages from the diet.

Chapter Five

Vulnerabilities

In this condition there is much damage that results to the blood-vascular system. By an astute practitioner this may be determined through serum tests. In fact, if severe, the adrenal case may prove to be anemic. The reference range will create confusion here. It is a physiological decline, and a reduction in the red cell count to less than ideal is an early warning sign. Full-fledged anemia is more rare but is an obvious sign. The hemoglobin may also be slightly reduced. As well, the total white count may be slightly or even moderately low. This is a sign of not only low adrenal output but also chronic fungal and/or viral infection. It is also a signal that the individual will be vulnerable to allergies and histamine response, as it is the function of these cells to deal with this.

Digestive disturbances are common. This is manifested predominately by vague digestive distress, heartburn, bloating, diarrhea, constipation, and even vomiting, the latter occurring only in extreme cases. Most commonly, the stool pattern alternates between diarrhea and constipation. Pebble-like stools are also typical. This may be the result of weakened intestinal motility from the lack of steroid production, or it can be the result of parasitic overload.

The individual may develop nerve-related signs such as tics, twitchings, sweaty palms, sweaty feet, and bizarre movements like contortions. Joint pain is common, especially in the upper back, mid-lower back, as well as the neck. There is usually constant stiffness of the neck and upper back. Often, sleep is impossible, even though the person is exhausted. There may be sleeping or napping on the job, a narcolepsy-like syndrome. There may also be difficult arising. The individual who sleeps till noon is typically Addisonian. There is muscular fatigue. The person with this condition might find it difficult to have the discipline for strenuous work. Yet, the most characteristic of all symptoms is the extreme tiredness with muscular weakness, a kind of worn-out, washed-out effect, often combined with obvious muscular fatigue. Addison claimed that a key in making the diagnosis is to determine if exhaustion is the main symptom, that is the symptom which has existed since the beginning of the condition.

Chronic state of dehydration?

The issue of salt and water balance as held by the body is a most serious issue. The human is not merely a bag of fluid; rather, such a one is filled with a saline solution. Any damage to the adrenal glands results in vast disruption of fluid dynamics. For instance, water balance can no longer be maintained; the person exists in a permanent state of dehydration. Salt is also impossible to properly retain, and thus, sodium deficiency is common and persistent. Excessive fluid consumption depletes it, as does a high potassium intake. For instance, potassium pills in adrenal types can prove catastrophic. This survival mode of attempting to conserve sodium explains the lack of thirst frequently encountered in adrenal cases.

This dehydration affects all tissues: there is a sort of dryness, even within the cells. The brain cells and spinal cord also become relatively dry. Thus, headaches, as well as stiff neck, are common. The stool dries up, and there is constipation. Drinking large amounts of water makes it worse by further depleting the sodium. Without this electrolyte in balance, water is lost through the urine. As the fluid levels drop further, weight loss may occur: blood pressure drops. The nervous tissues become further depleted, and the person becomes agitated. There may develop nausea and vomiting. Urine output declines; the urination may be in dribbles. If uncontrolled, this may lead to reactions such as shock or even death.

Dehydration may result in infection

Dry tissues, lack of blood volume, and dry membranes are a recipe for disaster. When the adrenals become damaged or infected, this results in an Addison's-like syndrome. For instance, tens of millions of Westerners suffer from defective, damaged, and infected adrenals. Thus, Addison's-like diseases are far more common that is realized.

The adrenals are vital to life. Moderate to severe damage to the glands always compromises the body. The usual result is failed organ function and/or serious disease. A list of diseases which result from damaged adrenals includes chronic fatigue syndrome, fibromyalgia, lupus, Crohn's disease, tuberculosis, diabetes, heart failure, asthma, viral syndrome, Epstein-Barr infection, leukemia, and systemic fungal infections. Also, numerous skin disorders may result, including hives, eczema, vitiligo, alopecia, and psoriasis. Other conditions which are related to weak or diseased adrenal glands include anxiety disorders, allergies, rhinitis, sinusitis, acne, and bronchitis.

Prior to the development of modern treatment Addison's was routinely fatal. On the short term artificial steroids seem to keep them alive, but there are numerous side effects. This includes joint/bone destruction. Then, it was discovered that an extract made from animal adrenal glands halted the crisis. Fishbein notes that hundreds of people who would otherwise have died were saved. Incredibly, the original treatments were natural extracts. These extracts have been systematically removed from the market by the drug powers.

Usually developing over a prolonged period, when it strikes with its usual ferocity, it gives the appearance of an acute illness. However, this is merely the final stage of a prolonged illness. The fact is the majority of Addison's victims fail to realize they have this condition until it is too late. What's more, physicians are wholly unaware of the early symptoms. Thus, they miss the diagnosis, usually deeming it as a psychological issue or stress. Or, they may diagnose some sort of disease, like GERD, migraine, hiatus hernia, esophagitis, spastic colon, yeast syndrome, chronic fatigue, fibromyalgia, depression, panic attacks, or similar vague illnesses, that disguises the cause. Yet, they never consider the real origin of these conditions, which is adrenal exhaustion.

The life and death function of the adrenals

It is no minor issue to have extremely weakened adrenal function. The weakness or exhaustion is typically from destructive dietary habits and also stress, although heavy exposure to vaccinations play a significant role. When these types of stresses are imposed upon them, these glands degenerate. This results in their infection by opportunists, especially TB and fungi. Now, they are incapacitated, and this is a potentially highly dangerous situation. The glands simply are incapable of producing sufficient cortisol to meet daily needs let alone those resulting from a crisis.

In fact, the adrenal type can die from sudden stress reactions. A life-threatening reaction may readily result, like anaphylactic shock or severe seizures. There can be sudden onset of pneumonia or other infections seemingly without explanation. Even so, it is important to realize the vulnerability. Another reaction could be heat shock or stroke, although this could also be related to other factors.

In untreated cases the infections can become overwhelming, leading to progressive disability, prostration, collapse, and death. These infections may not only be in the glands but also can develop systemically. Yet, no one knows they are occurring. No is medically assessed as having Addison's or, more correctly, sub-clinical Addison's syndrome with infection of the adrenal cortex, as symptoms are vague and diagnosed as another cause. Heartburn, vague digestive complaints, depression, anxiety, tiredness, irritability, weakness, barely able to function, and ultimately collapse: who will properly diagnose this as a type of Addision's disease? Instead, drugs are prescribed, including mood-altering ones, which conceal the symptoms. These also dangerously worsen the symptoms. This is why it is so crucial to achieve self-testing, as demonstrated by the following systematic approach.

Chapter Six

Testing Yourself

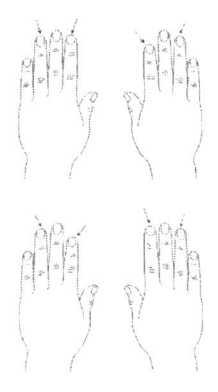

The symptoms and signs of adrenal collapse are well-published. Thus, self-testing is a reliable method for determining not only the existence of adrenal insufficiency but also its severity.

The following test will determine the degree of adrenal insufficiency. When taking this test, hand-held or desk mirror will be helpful.

Adrenal self-test (head)

Take the following test, adding one point per item, unless indicated otherwise. Which of these apply to you?

1. constant fatigue (3 points)
2. muscular weakness (2 points)

THE HEALTH BENEFITS OF ADRENAL METABO... 35

3. sweating or wetness of hands and feet (2 points)
4. nervousness or sensations of apprehension
5. insomnia (2 points)
6. very low blood pressure (3 points)
7. thin appearance of the face
8. hair is thin and wispy
9. chin is small, thin-boned, and/or receding (3 points)
10. dark or deep circles under the eyes
11. mood swings
12. paranoia
13. lightheaded sensation
14. cravings for salt (2 points)
—mild (2)
—moderate (3)
—extreme (4)
15. cravings for sugar
—mild (2)
—moderate (3)
—severe (4)
—extreme (6)
16. intolerance to fumes or cigarette smoke (2 points)
17. chronic stiffness of the neck or upper back (2 points)
18. hives and other rashes
19. vulnerable to food allergy reactions
20. generally weak; easily exhausted
21. get tired easily in the afternoon or after meals (2 points)
22. have no energy by the end of the day (2 points)
23. PMS
24. chronic heartburn
25. panic attacks (2 points)

26. unusually ticklish
27. hair loss on outer third of lower legs (2 points)
28. phobias
29. compulsive behavior
30. blood sugar disturbances
31. high sensitivity to noise (2 points)
32. easily frightened
33. easily frustrated
34. spastic neck
35. cold extremities
36. history of consuming large amounts of refined sugar (4 points)
37. run down (2 points)
38. weak voice (2 points)
39. weak heart or irregular pulse (palpitations)
40. easily distracted
41. tendency to have guilt feelings
42. clumsiness
43. skin has an unusual bronze color (3 points)
44. extremely sensitive to odors, perfume, and/or cigarette smoke (3 points)
45. crowding of the lower incisors (3 points)
46. first finger is longer than the ring finger
—on one hand (3 points)
—on two hands (4 points)
47. tendency to develop yeast or fungal infections
48. regularly use cortisone or prednisone or have used it heavily in the past (2 points)
49. pigment spots on temple, upper back, palm, lips, or chest (2 points)
50. easily develop lung or bronchial infections (2 points)

51. eczema and/or psoriasis
52. blond hair and blue-eyed
53. poor concentration (2 points)
54. depression
55. fainting spells (2 points)
56. unusually sensitive to smells (2 points)
57. history of food allergies
58. second toe is longer than the big toe (2 points)
59. constantly feel urge to urinate but volume is low
60. cravings for chocolate
61. all senses exceedingly acute (3 points)
62. nervous habit of rolling or twisting things (pillory)
63. vulnerable to viral infections, especially Epstein-Barr
64. loss of pigment on skin (vitiligo)
65. nervous habit of tapping the feet repeatedly

Your Score _____

Note: use the diagram, key signs, and the results of this test to make the most thorough and accurate assessment.

Anyone with a score above 7 has probable adrenal insufficiency, while a score from 10 to 16 indicates a mild-to-moderate case. A score from 17 to 24 indicates a moderate-to-severe case, while a score from 25 to 35 represents extreme adrenal exhaustion. A score from 36 to 42 is worrisome and represents profoundly extreme adrenal exhaustion, while any score above 40 is highly serious and represents the likelihood of potentially fatal adrenal collapse or at least the vulnerability for serious disease. Anyone who scores above 20 should be on a daily dose of the highly sophisticated naturally-produced cholesterol is the major lipid used in the synthesis of these hormones. Without it, the membranes of the cells degenerate.

Animal foods are the only dietary source of cholesterol. In fact, animals are synthetic factories for this substance. This is why for optimal hormonal balance the consumption of such foods is crucial. Thus, healthy sources of cholesterol—animal foods—must be included in the diet. These sources include organic whole milk, especially raw, unpasteurized, as well as yogurt, kefir, quark, and eggs. Other obvious sources include organ meats, red meat, poultry, seafood, and fatty fish. All such foods must be consumed from pure, unadulterated sources.

Adrenal-thyroid type

In this type there is a reversal of the hand sign seen in the thyroid-adrenal type. Here, on the dominant hand the adrenal sign predominates. For instance, if a person is right-handed, the index finger is longer than the ring or about equal with it, whereas on the opposite hand the thyroid sign, that is a short index finger compared to the ring, predominates (see Figures 8A and 8B). Another variation of this type is where both index fingers are nearly as long as the ring fingers. Usually, here, there is a higher score on the adrenal self-test than on the thyroid one.

The diet should be a combination of the foods recommended for adrenal and thyroid types. Coffee, tea, and chocolate should be avoided as well as white flour, commercial bread, and white rice. In particular, refined sugar must be strictly avoided. Usually, individuals with this type are intolerant to alcohol. Supplements include undiluted 3x royal jelly, wild sage, wild rosemary, natural-source vitamin C, whole food B complex powder, wild, remote-source kelp, raw purple maca, ashwagandha extract, and oregano juice. Unrefined sea salt should be used liberally in the diet.

Chapter Seven

Vaccination: aSerious Assault

Adrenal incapacitated individuals have a serious issue. They have weakened immunity. This is to the point where it may not even be competent. In this state it is easy for pathogens to colonize the individual. In essence with the dysfunctional adrenals they have virtually no resistance. After all, it is well-published that the chronic adrenal state is associated with infections by herpes, Epstein-Barr, candida, Lyme, and TB. The immune system is unable to overcome such invaders. In fact, any major, aggressive pathogen can gain a foothold.

There brings up the issue of the greatest toxin to all adrenal cases. This is vaccination, where live pathogens are injected into the body. This is a disaster for any adrenal case. In fact, the adrenal type has an extraordinarily high vulnerability for suffering vaccine reactions. It is an enormous risk not only for autism but also that of a host of other diseases. The conditions and syndromes that can be provoked in such cases include:

•juvenile rheumatoid arthritis

- leukemia
- diabetes type 1
- Hashimoto's disease
- chronic fatigue syndrome
- autism
- ADD
- Tourette's syndrome
- epilepsy
- Asperger's syndrome
- SIBO
- Crohn's disease
- spastic colon
- adrenal insufficiency
- salt-wasting syndrome

These are among the most disconcerting of all childhood diseases. An entire medical industry has been created surrounding these, and yet they are nearly entirely medically-induced. Make no mistake inoculations are a vast factor in the onset of adrenal syndromes. A person can only imagine the degree of stress placed on these glands by needles alone, which are completely anomalous for a newborn or infant. Without any strong immune development a high density of invasive microbes, infective DNA, human tissue components, and a litany of synthetic chemicals are injected. As a result, an enormous burden is placed upon the body which is well beyond the adrenal glands' capacities.

The adrenals are required to neutralize any toxic reaction. This is to such a degree that when the body is inoculated, it is these organs more than any other which are set into a reactionary phase. If they are strong enough, the person will survive. If not, there can not only be untoward reactions but also the onset of horrific childhood diseases, including especially type 1 diabetes, autism, juvenile rheumatoid arthritis, and cancer. With such a horrific immunological disruption there is even a risk for sudden death. This is hard evidence that the adrenals have no ability to compensate for this invasion.

Why assault them so severely? Why not simply let them be at peace as the develop through the natural means of development? The normal growth and development, matching or exceeding the standard charts—why not enjoy this while the child develops normally or even superiorly? To force their delicate and immature bodies into action through injecting deadly poisons via invasive procedures, is cruel at best. As a result, they develop diseases they would have never have contracted otherwise.

The adrenal syndrome creates the extreme vulnerability. This is demonstrated by the COVID-19 vaccine injury or death cases. Many of the individuals, who have suffered severe consequences, have low adrenal force. This is manifested by a number of the mentioned signs and symptoms, especially frail body structure, receding chin, crowding of the lower incisors, fine, wispy hair, low vocal capacity, and chronic weakness. When such people are injected, they are at a high risk for sudden death (see also www.cassingram.com). The coronavirus vaccines are a global disaster. Exceptionally deadly, in less than a half of a year as many as 250,000 Americans have died or have been permanently injured. Thousands of these cases were of the adrenal type and had little or no ability to combat the toxicity. Formulas and nutrients for detoxification include the oil of wild oregano, the wild oregano-based juice or essence, the whole, crude wild oregano herb with Mediterranean Sumac, the multiple spice oil complex, and the whole food vitamin C complex from wild camu camu plus acerola.

Chapter Eight

Conclusion

Adrenal insufficiency is a modern plague. Afflicting countless millions of people, it causes a wide range of symptoms and diseases. The mindless consumption of refined sugar is the bugaboo of humankind and certainly the primary factor leading to this disaster. Most people have no idea they have it, complicated by the fact that the symptoms are vague. Why is the individual so tired and weak? Why can't such a one handle stress? What is all this anxiety and depression about? Has anyone bothered to assess refined sugar consumption as the primary factor? This could be aggravated by a heavy intake of chocolate and caffeine. Is anyone evaluating this? If not, the tests on www.ebodytype.com could prove revealing.

Because of their symptoms they may be treated with medication that simply disguises the causes. For instance, there may be mood altering drugs prescribed for anxiety and depression, while sleep aids are taken for insomnia. Alcoholism may strike—the cravings could be overpowering—and there may be addiction to all manner of street drugs. The fact that the underlying factor for all these propensities is disturbed blood sugar is never considered.

Many may seek the care of psychiatrists for what is nothing other than a physical syndrome. As a result, they are prescribed mood-altering drugs, like Zoloft, Xanax, Effexor, and Paxil. Yet, there is no psychosis. Nor is there any degree of true depression or anxiety. The individual is merely deficient in adrenal steroids, while usually following a destructive diet.

The fatigue, weakness, irritability, and lack of concentration are "not in their heads" but, rather, are strictly the result of disturbed adrenal physiology. This is why it is so crucial to determine the type so all these can be diagnosed and properly treated. The headaches, muscular weakness, sweating of hands and feet plus the fact that they are ice-—none of these are worrisome conditions in themselves, as they are all explained as part of the adrenal syndrome.

It is ultra-important to determine the status. Which is it, adrenal, thyroid, pituitary, or thyroid-adrenal? Once this is achieved it is far easier to make the necessary adjustments. Now is the time to change any destructive ways. The negative thinking must be cleansed, while the psychic stress is minimized. These noxious emotions will deplete the glands, which may last for days and weeks and it is difficult to recover. In contrast, being happy and peaceful, being able to laugh in the heart no matter what will quickly revive them. The opposite, the dour and pessimistic, the negative and even obnoxious, will destroy them.

Categorically, the refined food must be eliminated or all will be naught. There is no way a person can continue to eat large amounts of refined sugar, processed starch, potatoes, and chocolate without suffering all manner of consequences. It is determined accurate that there is the adrenal component, which is either dominant or partial. It is also realized that this is driving most of the bad habits. So, now, it is easy. A person must eliminate the damaging food and noxious agents.

There will be no more refined sugar, white flour, white rice, commercial potatoes, fried food, or sugary drinks. It is a matter of survival. Nor will any stimulants be allowed: tobacco, energy drinks, cocoa, caffeine, and vanilla bean. Now, with all these major adjustments there will be no need for prescription drugs, and perhaps even those street drugs can be weaned off. For many people these will have to be slowly eliminated under a doctor's watch.

Alcohol is more of a depressant than a stimulant. Yet, it is nothing other than a refined carbohydrate, although it has the additional action of poisonous effects on the body. Like tobacco, it must be eliminated for the adrenals to recover.

There must be change, because this is in many cases a life or death matter. Otherwise, life will continue to be miserable and there could even be the development of disease syndromes. With diet alone and an increase in salt consumption there will be changes to the positive. Yet, this can be sped up by the intake of certain steroid-rich complexes. Premier among these are the triple strength royal jelly with wild rosemary and sage plus the ashwagandha 10:1 root extract concentrate. Another is the supplement complex containing New Zealand- or Argentinian-source grass-fed adrenal complex plus supportive herbs. This powerhouse formula must be relied upon for vigorous adrenal regeneration. The salt dose can be stabilized through the intake of the wild triple Salt Caps and also increased intake. The novel pine pollen powder, Mediterranean-source, may also proven invaluable, as, like royal jelly and ashwagandha, it is a rich source of steroids. Also available as sublingual drops in a black seed emulsion or a liquid drink formula these are potent formulas for reviving degenerated adrenal glands. As always, avoid all pollen supplements extracted in alcohol, in fact, any dietary supplements containing high concentrations of this adrenal poison.

The issue of TB and other fungal infection of the glands must always be addressed. In all sugar and chocolate addicts this is a highly likely consequence. This is where the juice of wild oregano is invaluable as is the oil. Use them to cleanse the TB and/or fungus out of the body. It takes about 90 days to do so. To do so the wild oregano therapy must be taken for at least a 90-day period. The steroid-containing supplements should be taken daily, as if like a replacement drug. These formulas include royal jelly with wild rosemary and sage, royal jelly-fortified ashwagandha, 10:1 extract, possibly, salt capsules, Mediterranean crude pine pollen, the adrenal health formula complex with Argentinian- or New Zealand-source beef glandulars. So must be increased salt intake. After countless years of abuse and neglect, plus toxicity, this will be sufficient to achieve adrenal regeneration and to maintain sound health of these glands.

About the Author

Cass Ingram is a nutritional physician who received a B.S. in biology and chemistry from the University of Northern Iowa (1979) and a D.O. from Des Moines Osteopathic College (1984). During medical school, he took a keen interest in the field of endocrinology. He often said that the endocrine system is **responsible for nearly every cell, organ, and function in the body, and should not be overlooked in the treatment of illness**. He kept this in mind while treating patients. In the 1980's he started the Arlington Preventive Medical Center in Arlington Heights Illinois, which later became the American Center for Curative Medicine. Ingram was a pioneer in the holistic and preventive medical field. In the early 1990's he stumbled upon wild oregano on a trip to his mother's home country of Lebanon, and after extensive research, he wrote the book" The Cure is in the Cupboard. . He has written over 25 books on natural healing and has given answers and hope to millions through interviews on thousands of radio and TV shows, as well as on his podcast 'The Wilderness Doc'. His research and writing have led to countless nature based cures and discoveries. Cass Ingram presents hundreds of health tips and insights in his many books on health, nutrition, and disease prevention. He promotes the curative properties of wild medicinal foods and spice extracts. For more information see purelywild.cassingram.com.

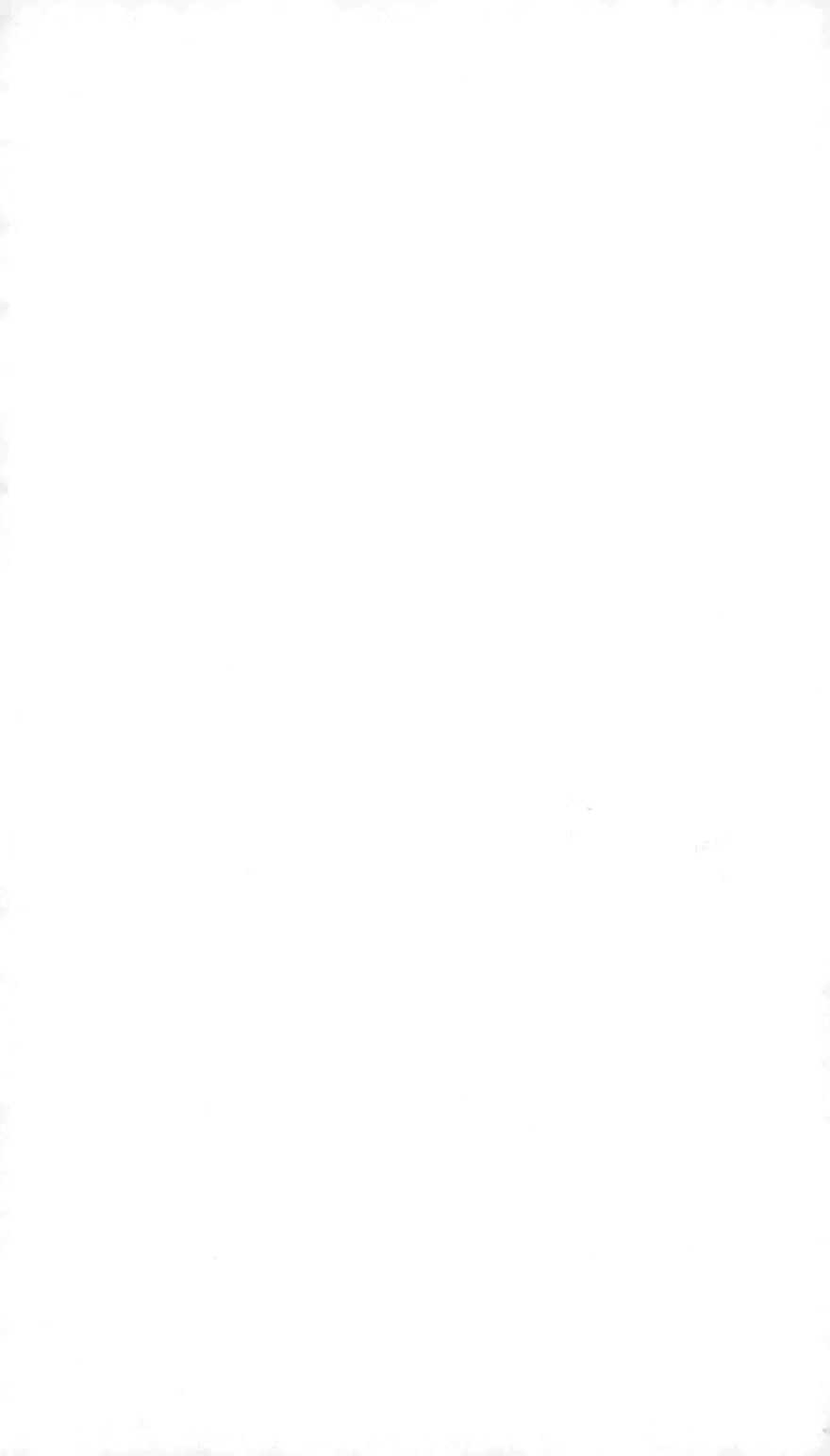

Made in the USA
Columbia, SC
06 January 2025